The Everyday Dash Diet Cookbook

Delicious Recipes to Lower Blood Pressure and Speed Weight Loss

Tom Connor

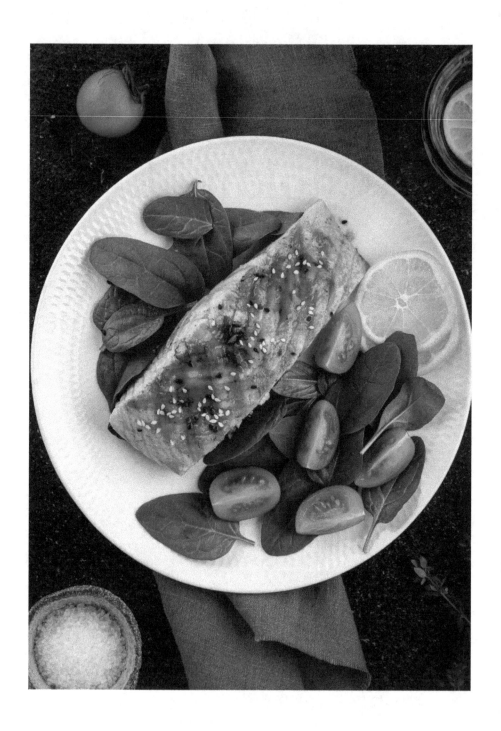

Contents

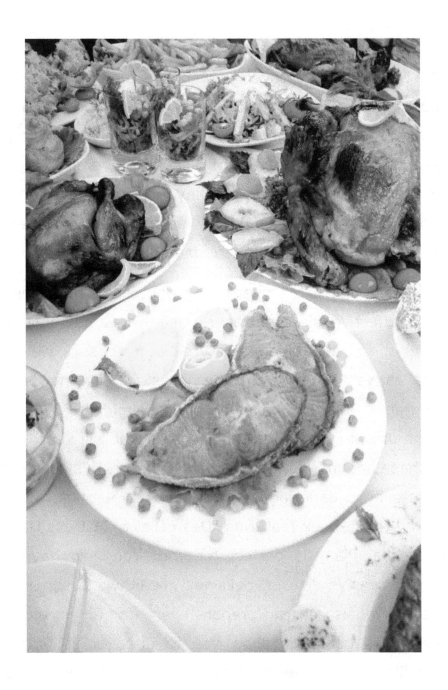

Introduction

The Dash Diet has proven to be one of the healthiest, most effective diets out there that have benefits in a lot of different health-related areas. From cancer to type 2 diabetes, from coronary heart disease to overall immunity enhancement and many more, diet-related problems. Dash diet has the power to prevent and even reverse some of the just mentioned diseases.

The Dash Diet has proven to be one of the healthiest, most effective diets out there that works not only to lower the body's blood pressure but to ensure weight loss, as well. When taking the first steps on a new diet program, however, it can be overwhelming to try and come up with meal ideas and recipes that will keep you in shape and in line with the diet. However, this does not have to be as daunting an experience as you think, which is why this e-book featuring "Dash Diet & 21 Days Dash Diet Meal Plan" is perfect for you. You now have a comprehensive list of delicious, healthy, Dash Diet-friendly meals you can prepare every day for an entire year! This book will allow you to discover all of the benefits of Dash Diet cooking and will even help you to discover some new meals that will quickly become your favorites.

DASH is an acronym for Dietary Approaches to Stop Hypertension, which was the name of the original study. The study organizers wanted to take the best elements of vegetarian diets, which were known to be associated with lower blood pressure, and design a plan that would be flexible enough to appeal to the vast majority of Americans, who are dedicated meat eaters. They developed what they believed was the healthiest omnivore diet plan. And the research has borne out this hope. The DASH diet helps lower blood pressure as well as the first-line medication for hypertension. It also lowers cholesterol. When evaluated over very long periods of time, the DASH eating pattern has been shown to help lower the risk for many diseases and life-threatening medical conditions or events, including stroke, heart attack, heart failure, type 2 diabetes, kidney disease, kidney stones, and some types of cancer. Not only is DASH recommended for people who have these conditions or are at risk for them, but it is recommended for everyone in the Dietary Guidelines for Americans. And the DASH diet is fabulous for weight loss, since it is loaded with bulky, filling fruits and vegetables and has plenty of protein to provide satiety.

Unfortunately, most people who are reading this book haven't noticed any major health problems as of yet, and their main concern is their current shape and how to make it better in a specific period of time. Fortunately for you, you will lose weight fast and naturally while following the Dash diet approach we represent in this book.

While still speaking about a perfect shape, it is also worth mentioning you will also be able to build lean mass and achieve any other fitness-oriented goal you want.

Along with meal plan, you will discover a huge variety of over 100 delicious Dash Diet recipes that will make you excited every time you cook or make your meal prep for the next days. Breakfast, lunch, dinner, various healthy snacks, and side-dishes will definitely satisfy your taste. And even if you have no previous cooking experience, this book also has recipes with less than 5 ingredients to start.

So don't wait, start your new healthy lifestyle right now!

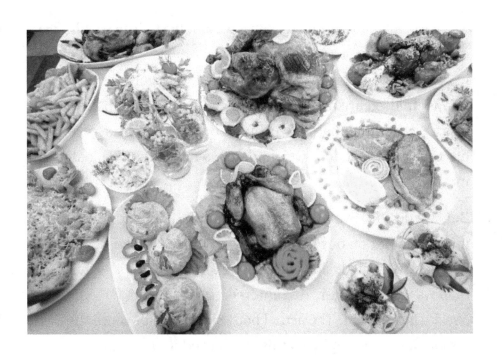

The Dash Diet

CHAPTER 1

The Psychology of Diet Preparation

Since we have numerous reasons, we resolve to lose weight: we don't like how we look, our clothes don't match, our wellbeing is in danger, the others are wandering, and our work is in danger, or our children are humiliated. We generally think about weight loss as something that only includes our body; definitely, no one has ever wanted to lose weight due to a fat brain or a bloated intellect.

But "we decide" is a function of the mind. It depends on our minds and not on our bodies when and why we take such a decision. We will decide whether we are five pounds heavier than we want, or after two hundred pounds and real medical obesity has passed. The actual body size does not cause the option of losing weight, as this is achieved in the brain.

Since the start (and follow-up) of a dietary program is a mental operation, it seems worth exploring what factors such decisions might cause.

1. Self-Image.

- one of us has a dual picture: our face to the world and our inner idea of how we look. Although we dress and groom to be seen by others as desirable, we are far less affected by others than by our satisfaction or disappointment with us.

Explore this idea by looking at yourself and others over the next week. You will find you are always complimented on the clothes you wear that you don't feel right. Wear a favorite costume perfectly suited, that you think looks amazing and that makes you particularly feel stirring - and nobody notices! The same thing happens with a hairstyle. One morning, you can't get your hair to do something, hurried for time, so you can pull it back with clips with frustration, and hope no one important is looking so bad. That's it! Three people say they like what you did with your hair.

When it comes to our weight, there is the same disconnect. When we look good in our eyes, we don't feel overweight, even though friends and colleagues gossip about our steady increase in weight. However, if we feel overweight, no reassurance from those around us will make us feel less fat. This mental image of our body size, taken to the extreme, can lead to anorexia Nervosa in eating disorders where excessively thin individuals keep their caloric intake dangerously reduced because they constantly feel too large.

We then decide to take a diet in response to our internal self-image. Some of the advantages that we expect are lean and fit take into account others: I'll be more attractive to the opposite sex; I will be noted when it comes to promotion at work; my family and friends will be jealous and have to reassess me as a stronger person than they thought. But what it does for us individually is the true incentive for getting in shape. It is the need to feel better about ourselves, which leads us to diet and exercise through pain and Monotony. It is the vision of us in the future that leads us to our target. Losing this hope or concluding, we won't feel that much better about ourselves are the reasons we give up and slip into the relative convenience of "okay." settling.

2. Body versus Mind dominance.

We all fight for a lifelong inner struggle between our mind and body. Each stage of development is dominant. As kids, we are just a series of sensations. We discover the exciting new world around us by touching everything within reach, sampling everything we can put in our mouths, looking around at the gestures and all the sounds we hear, until finally, we learn to mimic them.

When we step into our early years of education, we begin to reflect on our minds. We eat vast quantities of knowledge voraciously. We learn to read, and our planet extends its borders by 1000 percent. We learn to use the internet, and we have an infinite world at hand.

Then we pass into puberty, and our beauty becomes the primary factor of daily life overnight. We sail through the pitfalls and joys of adolescence, where success and coolness are much more important than learning or mental growth. We spend a very long time on our bodies. We're trying new clothing, new hairstyles, and new maquillage. We have pierced body parts and are exposed to tattoo discomfort because it would make us stand out. We primp, groom, and push ourselves into the models that have been judged by our peers as in."

When we mature, we aspire to reconcile our physical and mental selves. While our corps is supreme in the world of attracting one, we need to practice our minds to advance our careers and establish deep relationships that go far beyond physical attraction.

When we settle down and start creating the good life we want, our energies and efforts turn to things outside of us: children, significant others, friends, family, and jobs. We have so much going on around us that we lose contact with our bodies and minds. We fall into our own comfort zone where food meets so much of our needs. It eases our tension, alleviates our daily tensions, and makes constant blues endurable. It eats away our social connections. It becomes a crucial part of how we express love for those we love. We always see ourselves as we once were and ignore the love handles and pockets of fat that we strongly overlook parts of our body. Our bodies and our inner image of our bodies are becoming increasingly discordant.

3. Our sense of self-efficacy.

Self-efficacy is a psychological concept to describe the perception of a person that any action they take influences the outcome. It is neither self-confidence nor the assumption that you are capable of doing something, although it can include both. It represents our inner hope that what we do will bring about our desired results.

If we begin a diet, want to shape, or begin to take better care of ourselves is essentially a personal choice that may or may not is made as we have expected. The difference lies in the assumption of success, and it's always easier to go on a path that we expect to be successful than to travel to a target where disappointment is the most likely result.

How do we incorporate these principles to make us lean, healthy, and attractive?

We start by looking at our self-image and how we appear to others. Only telling someone Do you think I'm getting too heavy?" does not work unless you have a brutally frank friend or ask somebody who you don't like. Most of us are culturally trained to save the feelings of others so that the answers to such a question are more respectful than real.

Specific focusing can provide better feedback. Tell others that you have a survey for a class you take. Offer a short one-page questionnaire that allows any friend or colleague to list three adjectives that identify various aspects of your physical appearance. Complete yourself one of the sheets. Make sure the responses are confidential by demanding that no names be used and that someone else gathers the sheets completed.

Once the answers are available, compare them to your own answers and see where the descriptions are different. You might find yourself a little defensive. It's not an exercise to make you feel bad about yourself or to gloat about the unexpected compliments. It is an orchestrated endeavor to help you assess the distance between your self-image and your image in the world. Those areas of divergence are a starting point to overlap the two photos.

After defining areas of work, it is time to draw on the unmistakable power of our wonderful mind to start imposing the structure and organization, which we will have to introduce the desired changes. Our mind can only take us where we want to go if it is supported by confidence in our ability to achieve success. Now is the time to reject any failure expectations. Many failed diet and exercise attempts have been made in the past. Leave the past. Leave the past. We are not destined to continue unproductive behavior. We have the gem of a creation, the human mind, able to do almost everything. If we concentrate on any mission, it will succeed if our concerns and doubts do not interfere.

By exploring our memories, we draw on our optimistic aspirations to build up a long list of past achievements. There can be big benchmarks such as endorsing a campaign we liked, planning a great event, or establishing an intense relationship with ourselves. The smallest personal victories are, however, the most important but are generally easily overlooked or dismissed.

Studies and a strong degree in a challenging class show clearly the ability to produce the results you want. Go for quantity: the day you grinned over someone in a smoky room and finished with a short but beautiful affair; the timing study that no-one expected; the night you spin on ice skates. Continue: make the drill squad, shoot a stolen basket, make your own promotional outfit, dying in a wonderful color in your own bathroom, catch a ball, find new apps on your machine and burn your first CD. The list can be infinite and will linger while you recall snippets of the past that you have been burying for a long time.

Hold this list close and read it on a regular basis. It's your self-effective pep band.

You now know the fields in which you can operate and trust the success of your efforts. You must now identify the internal benefits that good weight loss brings. Feel strong, enjoy step-by-step, and quickly zipping your clothes are quick starters. Unconsciously heading to the pool in a short suit is a fantasy enhancing. Making a sales success with the belief that you look best is a picture you will appreciate as you fall asleep. Having someone you like admires or seeing your rivals, jealously emphasizes your determination and maintains the inconvenience of dieting and the demands of repetitive workout routines.

You know where you are going, you know what it will take, and you know that you will succeed. Your mind is set, just waiting for your decision day. Whenever you choose, you will make a choice because you are now under power.

What is Dash Diet Eating Plan?

The dietary eating plan DASH (Dietary Methods to Stop Hypertension) is one of the non-pharmacological therapies for controlling blood pressure. This involves dietary improvements, which include: low consumption of saturated fat, increased fruit and vegetable intakes, more replaced carbohydrate-containing foods, such as whole-grain products, increased seafood, poultry, and nuts intake. The study has shown that the nutritional plan for DASH has the highest effect on blood pressure and cholesterol reduction compared to normal diets. The result is evident within two weeks!

Downward Calory Tips Intake With DASH Eating Schedule!

1. Increase fruit

An apple holds the doctor away for one day! In the food plan for high blood pressure patients, apple and dried apricots are the best options.

2.Growth of vegetables

Burger! Yes, your blood pressure may increase, even if it's a favorite food for most people. I know it's really difficult for you to avoid eating it. However, I recommend that you weigh 3 ounces of meat rather than 6 ounces in the larger size.

The same goes for limiting chicken consumption by just 2 ounces and with a plate of raw vegetables.

3.Enhance fat-free or fat-free dairy products

For example, common ice cream can be replaced with low-fat yogurt.

Reducing Salts and Sodium

By ingesting more fruit and vegetables in the DASH food plan, the lower amount of sodium has made it possible to consume less salt and sodium. Furthermore, fruit and vegetables are rich in potassium and play a part in lowering high blood pressure. Milk products and fish are other important dietary sources.

Tips for Salt and Sodium Reduction

Restrict food high in salt. It is safer to eat no or low-salt foods.

Increased vegetable consumption.

No salted rice, pasta, or other mixed foods

Remove extra salt from preserved foods, such as tuna or beans preserved in a can.

Dash Diet Eating Plan

What is the food for DASH? The DASH diet literally means nutritional methods to avoid high blood pressure. In the early stages of high blood pressure, people are frequently put on this diet to help regulate blood pressure.

The plan is focused on 2,000 calories a day but can be changed to suit your nutritional needs. The American Heart Association recommends this diet highly because it helps to achieve excellent health in many other ways than hypertension. The most significant ingredients to naturally support hypertension are foods high in potassium, foods with calcium and magnesium.

First of all, the DASH strategy assigns great importance to crops. It is good to add whole wheat pieces of bread, wheat pastes, and whole-grain cereals with 7-8 portions per day as a daily allowance on this schedule. Your whole grain has far more nutritional qualities than those that have more refined sugars.

The DASH diet plan also encourages fruit and vegetables. You must eat four to five portions of this category every day. As you review the DASH diet guide, the author tells you several ways to include your regular servings of fruits and vegetables.

Next to this plan are non-fat and low-fat dairy products. You will have to select skim milk, or at most 1 percent, low fat or unfat cheeses and yogurts.

You have lean meat options after milk. There are small portion sizes, indicating no more than two parts. Healthy options include low-fat frankfurters, skinless chicken, and other meat.

When you come to the section where nuts and seeds are listed, they are permitted but are restricted to only five small portions a week. This included legumes as well.

The plan book on the DASH diet is complete. Since you need the plan to fit your everyday calories, it will show you how. This book will also teach you about healthy ways to eat. Eating out is a real challenge in a diet, but the DASH diet book shows you how.

The strategy contains a portion of the book on workouts and alcoholic drinks as well as ways to help you get out of smoking habits.

Additional medical issues with insulin resistance, cholesterol, and inflammation tend to be beneficial. If you have some of these other medical conditions than hypertension, you should like this meal plan very much.

What You Need To Know About The DASH Diet
Our foods will affect our overall health. A diet rich in unhealthy components such as saturated fats and cholesterol is a healthy way to achieve high blood pressure and other diseases. On the other hand, the right food option will reduce the risk of contracting these diseases.

There is a specific eating plan which has demonstrated lower blood pressure or hypertension. This diet is known as DASH or Nutritional Stop Hypertension Approaches.

The DASH diet was a product of clinical trials performed by scientists from the NHLBI. Researchers have found that a diet that is high in potassium, magnesium, calcium, protein, and fibre and low in fat and cholesterol can reduce high blood pressure significantly.

The study showed that even a diet rich in fruits, vegetables, and low-fat milk products has a major influence on hypertension reduction. It also showed that the DASH diet results easily, often in just two weeks from the beginning of the diet.

Three essential nutrients are also stressed by the DASH diet: magnesium, calcium, and potassium. These minerals are intended to minimize hypertension. A standard 2000-calorie diet includes 500 mg of magnesium, 4,7 g of potassium, and 1,2 g of calcium.

Doing the DASH Diet

It is very easy to follow the DASH diet and takes a little time to pick and prepare meals. Foods high in cholesterol and fats are stopped. Dieters should eat as much as possible of vegetables, fruits, and cereals.

Because the foods you consume in a DASH diet are high in fiber content, you can slowly increase your fiber-rich food intake to help prevent diarrhea and other digestive problems. By consuming an additional portion of fruit and vegetables with every meal, you will steadily increase your fiber intake.

Grains are also healthy sources of fiber and vitamins, and minerals of the B-complex. Whole grains, whole wheat bread, bran, wheat germs, and low-fat cereal are all grain items that you can consume to improve your intake of fiber.

You can select the food you consume by looking at processed and packaged food product labels. Check for low-fat, saturated fat, sodium, and cholesterol foods. The main source of fat and cholesterol is meat, chocolates, chips, and fast snacks, so you can limit your intake of such products.

If you wish to eat meat, limit your meal to just six ounces a day, which is close in size to a card deck. In your meat dishes, you should eat more fruits, cereals, pasta, and beans. Often a large protein source without excess fat and cholesterol is low-fat milk or skim milk.

You can taste both canned or dried fruit and fresh fruit for snacks. Snack choices are also available to those on the DASH diet, including graham crackers, unsalted nuts, and fatty yogurt.

It's Easy to DASH

It is popular with many health buffs, as no special meals and recipes are required. There are no special preparations and calorie counting as long as you eat more fruits and vegetables and reduce the consumption of foods high in fat and cholesterol.

The DASH diet is the balanced diet that focuses more on the three main minerals, which are expected to have a beneficial impact on high blood pressure.

The DASH diet is perfect for people who enjoy eating comfort and convenience. The DASH diet provides tried and tested dietary systems for people who aim for good health with empirical evidence to support them.

CHAPTER 2

5 Benefits of a DASH Diet - Proven to Lower Your Blood Pressure

Tracking your diet is a good way of life, and it helps you to check your medical condition. Many common dietary regimes can be practiced, and the DASH diet is one of them.

DASH has been shown to reduce blood pressure levels.> It was created for hypertensive people by adopting a soft or salty food plan with minimum saturated fats and cholesterol. It is not meant for those who want to lose weight, but it is also possible to do certain workouts by decreasing calorie intake.

DASH has five advantages to deliver if strictly observed. The first is to decrease body weight, saturated fat, and cholesterol. This will avoid a heart attack, stroke, and other cardiovascular diseases.

Secondly, the increased consumption of lycopene, beta-carotene, and phytochemicals in the body is also increased by fruits, vegetables, and low-fat milk products. Phytochemicals help protect the body against cardiac cancer and disease in plants.

Third, the consumption of fiber is increased by the inclusion of whole grain items in the plan. Fiber helps to absorb food and to reduce cholesterol levels.

Fourthly, sodium decreases in one's diet to a maximum of 1.500 mg per day can be an effective hypertension treatment. The less salt ingestion, the lower the blood pressure. The risk of atherosclerosis and congestive cardiac insufficiency is thus decreased.

Fifthly, high sugar candy and drinks are avoided. This helps to reduce the consumption of calories and preserves the body's sugar balance.

In short, DASH's diet includes minerals such as magnesium, potassium, calcium, and protein. It not only decreases sodium and cholesterol in the body but also provides the main body nutrients required.

The DASH Diet: Does It Work?

Maybe you learned of the Hypertension DASH Diet.

Well, it is now one of the most well-known diet plans in the world and can be more than a trend. Built by the National Institutes of Health of the Department of Health and Human Services, this diet program is focused on nutritional facts.

DASH is an acronym for Dietary Approaches to Hypertension Stop, which essentially shows how the food you consume will reduce your blood pressure. The premise of the diet is to instruct men and women with high blood pressure and high blood pressure on how to eat much better and minimize blood pressure and connected diseases. High blood pressure is also an issue that can potentially be prevented with a safe way of living, but it can only be handled if a person has it.

Elevated blood pressure is serious and can also lead to coronary artery disease, dementia, stroke, and finally, cardiac failure. Figure that about 33% of men and women actually have high blood pressure or high blood pressure. It is one-third of the adult population, so it is possible that you or someone you know will be diagnosed as having the disease.

The DASH Hypertension Diet will help you to reduce your blood pressure and risk of affiliated diseases by laying down a few guidelines. For example, one of the key guidelines set out in the weight loss plan is to cut the intake of sodium to between 2.300 and 1.500 mg per day. This can look like you still get a lot of sodium, but not so much, in fact.

Consider some of the things that you might eat every day...

Did you know that a fourth pound of cheese contains around 1,190 milligrams of sodium? This is practically the whole daily allowance if you restrict yourself to 1,500 mg a day. Even at 2,300 a day, the proposed daily portion is still over 50 percent.

And if you believe you will be mindful of your health and receive salad, be warned... Condiments and dressings have become infamous for large sodium levels.

So, what are you going to get into the DASH Diet?

A lot of fruit and vegetables per day instead of sweets and desserts

Foods rich in fiber as an alternative to processed carbs

Low fat and fat-free milk products, not whole milk products

Water and soda club in relation to sugar soft drinks

The DASH Diet is not only a nutritional agenda; it also advises on safe lifestyles:

Join a workout, whether the blood pressure level is typical or not.

Try in doing at least 30 minutes of exercise every day.

Determine your own weight loss goals

If you take high blood pressure prescription medications, do not forget to take them every day.

It's no wonder with such common-sense recommendations that the DASH Diet is at present gaining such popularity. This is a meaningful diet that gives you the ability to lose weight and stay healthy. And people with healthy blood pressure will generally benefit from a DASH diet and adhere to a high fiber, low-fat, reduced-sodium diet. If you adopt this diet, you can not only shed pounds, and it can potentially save your lives.

The Best Diabetes Diet - The DASH Diet

Over time a large number of diabetes diets have been developed; that is to say, diets developed to enhance diabetes control have developed, have a heyday and sunny retirement. However, many remain strong and as successful as they were initially introduced. But how effective these diets are, exactly.

With the list seemingly rising by the year, a frustrated public sometimes wonders where to start. I, therefore, wanted to review the most common diets on the market at the moment, and at the conclusion of this review, two diets were established as excellent performers to support people with diabetes. One of them is the diet of DASH. The following is a short description of what I heard about this diet. But before we get into it, you might want to ask, what is a healthy diabetic diet exactly? Therefore the following are only some of these elements.

It is low in carbohydrates or at least provides a way to even out the carbohydrate during the day or to "burning" excess, as in the case of exercise.

It should be rich in dietary fiber and has demonstrated several health benefits, such as a low glycemic index and a decrease in probabilities of heart disease, etc.

Low salt. Salt low. Salt can lead to high blood pressure, so it is important to reduce it.

Low in fat. Low in fat. Since foods or fat easily converted to fat like sugar can lead to overweight of the person – a risk factor for diabetes, such foods often need low-fat content.

A healthy diabetic diet should aim to achieve the recommended daily potassium allowance. Potassium is important because it could help to reverse the adverse effects of salt on the circulatory system.

Obviously, the DASH diet has all these features and more. Yet just what the DASH diet is and how it happened. Well, the DASH Diet was created in 1992, which means nutritional methods to avoid hypertension. Under the aegis of the United States. The National Heart, Lung and Blood Institute, National Institute of Health (NIS), and five of the best-respected health centers in the United States have collaborated to study the impact of diet on blood pressure. As a result of this study, the DASH diet, the best diet for balanced blood pressure, was formulated.

But this is not as far as its advantages are concerned. The diet was also found to be as good as a diabetes diet. In reality, in the 35 diets analyzed by US News and the World report earlier this year, the Biggest Loser Diet was the best diet for diabetes. In addition to the guidance given by the American Diabetes Association, both the prevention and control qualities of diabetes were shown.

Prevention has proven that it helps people lose weight and even holds them away. As overweight is a significant risk factor for developing type 2 diabetes, it is a diabetes dietary preference.

Furthermore, a combination of the DASH diet and calorie restrictions reduces the risk factors associated with metabolic syndrome, which raises the likelihood of developing diabetes. Regarding regulation, the findings of a small study published in the 2011 edition of Diabetes Care showed that DASH type 2 diabetics had decreased A1C levels and their fasting blood sugar for eight weeks.

Moreover, the diet was found to be more versatile than most, which makes it easier to follow and adapt to encourage the patient to follow a doctor's dietary advice.

Another advantage of this diet is its compliance with dietary guidelines. Bright, as it might seem, this is actually very important since certain diets limit certain foods, leaving the person in certain nutrients and minerals potentially deficient.

A summary of this conformity reveals that the fat diet is satisfyingly below the 20 to 35% of the government-recommended daily calories. It also reaches the 10% overall saturated fat threshold, which falls just below that. The recommended amount of proteins and carbohydrates is also met.

For salt, the guideline has meal limits for this mineral. Both the recommended daily maximum of 2,300 mg and the AU maximum of 1,500 mg if you are 51 years of age or older or have hypertension, diabetes, or chronic kidney disease.

This diet also properly takes care of other nutrients. This diet offers a strong supply of the recommended daily intake of 22 to 34 grams of fiber for adults. Even potassium, a nutrient characterized by its ability to prevent salts, raises blood pressure, decreases the risk of developing renal stones, and also reduces bone loss. Impressively because of the difficulty in getting the recommended daily intake of 4,700 mg or 11 bananas a day.

The minimum daily intake of vitamin D is penciled at 15 mg for adults who are not getting enough sunlight. Although the diet is just shy of this, it is proposed that vitamin D fortified cereal can easily be made up of.

Calcium is also properly treated by the diet for healthy bones and teeth, blood vessel development, and muscle function. The guideline of the government between 1,000 mg and 1300 mg can easily be met without any air or grace. The same applies to vitamin B-12. The recommendation of the government is 2.4 mg. The supply of diets is 6.7.

From the above, it can be seen that the DASH diet is an excellent option in choosing a diet that will help you control your diabetes. While it is the second-largest loser in this diet, it has the advantage of being specially formulated to help lower blood pressure and is equally effective in this regard. So the DASH diet is highly recommended if you are searching for a great diabetes diet.

Type 2 Diabetes - The DASH Diet and Gestational Diabetes

Much as one health issue sometimes leads to another, improvements in a healthier lifestyle can often fix more than one health problem. The British Journal of Nutrition published a study on dietary approaches to avoid hypertension in gestational diabetes in November 2012.

Researchers have studied 34 female gestational diabetes diagnosed at 24 to 28 weeks of pregnancy. Seventeen women remained in daily diets of 45% to 55% carbohydrates, 15% to 20% protein, and 25% to 30% total fat, and 17 others with the DASH diet.

This diet has been similar to normal diets but has increased fruit, vegetables, whole grains, and fatty milk products and less cholesterol, saturated fat, salt, and refined grains.

After four weeks, the women showed on the DASH diet:

- •lower blood pressure
- •lowered HbA1c levels
- Improved blood sugar levels

That at the start of the analysis. The cholesterol in these women was also lower than in the normal diet.

The DASH diet has inferred from these findings that the tolerance to sugar and blood cholesterol of women with gestational diabetes is beneficial in comparison with the normal diet.

The DASH diet was intended to regulate high blood pressure by having a lifelong diet that is low in sodium chloride or table salt. Vegan diets have proven to be the best kind for diabetes, but people with diabetes will consume most of the DASH diet prescribed.

- 4 to 5 portions of fruit are recommended per day, either for desserts or between meals. Leave on the peels to provide fiber, vitamins, and texture whenever possible.
- 4 to 5 portions of vegetables on this diet are also recommended.
- Also recommended are 6 to 8 parts of whole grains.
- Tofu plates can be supplemented with 6-8 servings of DASH meat.
- We also suggest 4 to 5 portions of nuts and beans a week.
- 2 to 3 portions of oil are in the diet, with the best types of liquid oils like olive, soy, or canola.
- 5 or fewer sweet portions are recommended.

The DASH diet advises that men and women can restrict alcoholic drinks to 1 or 2 daily. Caffeine is non-commitment, but many doctors agree that caffeine is not a good option during pregnancy.

Both hypertension and gestational diabetes are conditions that can be stopped during pregnancy. Isn't it nice to help keep both health issues away from a balanced diet?

Type 2 diabetes is just not a disease with which you have to deal with. It doesn't have to get worse slowly and eventually. You can control the disease: start with a healthy diet and recover your health.

CHAPTER 3

8 Advisable Foods While on a DASH Diet - Save Your Body From High Blood Pressure

The nutritional methods to avoid hypertension or DASH have been established with a set of approaches for people who want to regulate their starved behaviors in order to lessen the dangers of high anxiety levels. It is also useful for the defense of diets against osteoporosis and common human diseases such as stroke, cancer, diabetes, and heart failure. Save yourself from multiple risks of hypertension; use the eight foods you should consume for a dietary approach.

1. Grains supply healthy sources of nutrition in the body, enriched with whole grains, such as pieces of bread, cereals, oatmeal, pasta, and rice.

2. Fruits and vegetables - These two foods, eight to ten servings each, are recommended for daily consumption. Fiber, protein, carbohydrates, vitamins, and minerals are rich in tomatoes, carrots, broccoli, and sweet potatoes, as well as bananas, apes, and prunes.

3. Dairy products — The three primary dairy enterprises supplying major vitamins, calcium, and protein are milk, yogurt, and cheese. During the DASH reduction, fat-free or low-fat milk products are successful.

4. Meat, poultry, and fish—meat and fish are rich in protein, vitamin-B, iron, and zinc, whether refined or untreated. Prepare and cook correctly before broiling, roasting, or frying, taking the skin and fats.

5. The almonds, kidney beans as well as sunflower seeds, and the like are healthy magnesium, potassium, and protein source. They are also rich in fiber and help to battle cancers and cardiovascular diseases through their phytochemicals.

6. Fats and oils-fat enriched diets help the organism consume important immune vitamins; the risk of cardiovascular disease, diabetes, and obesity may be amplified by excessive fats.

7. Low-fat Sweets — In this program, jellybeans, graham crackers, and light-flavored cookies are also considered for consumption. Dark chocolate is recommended as it contains fewer hypertensive substances.

8. Snacks with low sodium—buy foods that have "no salt added" or logos of the "low sodium-rich" found in bold sections of the snack.

Now you want more energy, healthiness, look younger, weight loss, and body washing, right?

DASH Diet Plan - The Key to Lower Blood Pressure

Which ones would you prefer to regulate your high blood pressure, take costly medications with nasty side effects every day or turn to a proven diet that can help normalize your blood pressure in around two weeks?

It sounds stupid, but millions of people choose to take blood pressure medicine when they can improve their condition by adapting their DASH diet as part of their cure.

The Dietary Approach to Stop Hypertension (DASH) is a diet intended to minimize blood pressure. Contrary to fad weight-loss diets, it is not impossible to adhere to and has huge advantages not only in controlling blood pressure but also in reducing the chances of other diseases such as diabetes and cancer.

Diet plays a significant role in both developing and reducing high blood pressure. Food is the power of our body. When you take a minute to think, a bad diet is just like pouring gas into a tank, which runs unleaded. The engine will still operate, but it will run approximately and simply stop working overtime because of the build-up of fuel. A load of salt, sugar, and saturated fat on our bodies has the same effect.

There are two explanations for why the DASH diet plan works. Second, it consists of foods rich in vitamins, minerals, fibers, and antioxidants that lower pressure and reverse blood harm. Secondly, and just as critically, it substitutes for the junk that caused the problem.

Here are the types of foods you can expect from the DASH diet quickly:

- Whole grains, such as cereals, oatmeal, and whole-grain bread, deliver complex carbon and fiber products.
- Fruits such as spinach, tomatoes, bananas, beans, and berries, which supply potassium, magnesium, fibre, and antioxidants.
- No oily or fatty dairy products such as fatty milk, yogurt, and cheese that supply protein, calcium, and magnesium.
- Magnesium and Protein lean poultry, white meats, and fish.
- Nuts seeds and beans such as kidney beans, almonds and calcium, fiber, and vitamin B pistachios.
- Nice fats and oils like canola oil, olives, and our fats avocados.

It takes the diet to make it work, and it will take some plans, particularly for the food you eat. However, compare this piece of work to the prescription for drudgery and pain, and I hope you're sure that it's worth the effort.

In less than two weeks, your blood pressure reading can drop by 20 points following the DASH diet plan, combined with a bit of daily exercise and relaxation technique. Give it a chance; give it a try. Your heart's going to thank you.

The DASH diet - Foods to avoid

In this section, let us quickly look at the Dash Diet menu and see if it's all cracked up - and if our New Years' weight loss targets can be reached if we comply!

The nutritional solution to avoid a high DASH diet is a weight loss strategy tailored for moderate and sensitive eating. This method is increasingly popular as it focuses on an approach to healthy eating in the real world. Indeed, you can eat and enjoy yourself without having to count any calories in your diet if you obey their suggestion. Quick food is also OK for road warriors with this varied diet approach. Some restaurants also support dieticians using symbols on the menus to classify low-fat items. Diners are also given more room to choose how to prepare their meals.

Research suggests that this mix of nutrients can decrease blood pressure. DASH may also lead to reducing the risk of chronic disease and maintaining a balanced and healthy weight.

The DASH diet encourages cholesterol- and saturated fat-low foods. Cutting fatback is OK to retain the taste of healthy food and a choice menu. Here are some main ingredients for your success with this very common approach.

1) If you can, stay away from the bread, but when you're too hungry and the rolls on the table are too tenting - Well - just don't use butter.

2) To salad dress- ask for low fat on one side and on the other side.

3) Choose the green or spinach tossed

4) Ask your food to be prepared instead of butter with olive oil.

5) The foods that are steamed, broiled, grilled, roasted, or stir-fried should be picked.

6) Choose vegetables as the side dishes. Baked potatoes and rice are also all right.

7) Skip onion rings and French fries

8) Cut off any obvious meat fat.

9) Drinking water, soda club, juice, dietary soda, tea, or coffee is healthier

10) Say no to booze too much! (Be limited to two)

13) Skip soup and choose fruit or salad instead.

14) Always be mindful of salt consumption!

And naturally...the law of the jumbo scale is coming next!

15) Always stop too much to eat!

Other aspects the DASH diet points out are more evident pitfalls that dieters fall into the Salad paradox... Do not only assume that it has green, and it's safe or low in calories - certain dressings of salad are fat, fat, FATTENING!

A smart approach to dieting, but it won't revolutionize your figure or turn you easily into a hard body. But if you want to be just a little healthier and self-conscious, this is a small but necessary step in the correct direction!

The DASH Diet Could Help In The Fight Against Obesity

Like it or not, obesity is the first line of attacks in the conventional diet and exercise plan, and most doctors don't even recommend stomach bypass surgery until they are confident that you have actively and successfully attempted to diet and exercise. In the face of having to walk along a dietary path, it makes sense to select a diet that is at least able to function.

One potential alternative is the DASH diet, ultimately formulated to lead to lower blood pressure and endorsed by the National Heart, Lung and Blood Institute and the American Heart Association.

Many diets concentrate on foods that you should avoid, for example, that require you to cut carbohydrates or fats. Others concentrate on the nutritional properties of such foods and require you to eat massive amounts of items such as grapefruit. Without getting into the inside and outside of these diets, the real issue is that they have been shown to be unsuccessful time and time again. Simply put - they're not working.

So what is the difference in the DASH diet?

The DASH diet focuses on what to eat rather than what to eat and advises the simplest thing to eat the fruit and vegetable mix balanced with some low-fat dairy items.

Over two main factors, fruit and vegetables are excellent dietary items (as long as you eat a variety of both products and do not only limit yourself to one or two of your favorite products).

First of all, fruit and vegetables are high in water and low in calories. This means you don't have to eat huge amounts either to feel satisfied, and even relatively large amounts don't offer a high-calorie intake.

Second, fruits and vegetables not only provide your adequate daily intake of fiber but also provide essential vitamins and minerals that are necessary for healthy eating.

Whether or not the particular DASH diet is a personal preference, but when you have to try a diet and practice a solution to obesity, it could be an excellent route to take a diet which complies with the concepts outlined in the DASH diet and which mainly focuses on fruit and vegetables.

Heart Healthy Foods

The National Heart, Lung, and Blood Institute and the American Heart Association support DASH's heart-healthy diet. DASH stands for (Dietary Hypertension Avoid Approaches). It is also the base of the current USDA MyPyramid. The basis of the DASH diet is obviously nothing new for you. This includes berries, vegetables, whole grains, and fats that are low in saturation. "It's not glamorous" Learn more about the new and improved diet that is safe at heart, and did I mention it will help to protect against cancer and undesired weight?

The basis of a balanced heart diet is:

Total fat: 27%

Saturated fat: 6%

Protein: 18%...

Carbohydrates: 55%

It also contains not more than 2300 mg (1500 mg is better) of sodium per day and at least 30 g of fiber. This means very little for you if you're like me and you'd rather only know what foods to consume and which foods to avoid. So, I'm going to put the DASH diet on your base shelf.

Eating Foods:

It is essential for oily fish and/or lean protein. Salmon, tuna, and mackerel are plentiful in omega-3 fatty acids, which have been shown to enhance the elasticity of your blood vessels. Chicken and turkey breast are always good protein choices if fish isn't your solid.

Fruit and vegetables were high in antioxidants that protect the blood vessels from heart disease through neutralizing damaging free radicals. It is an established way to help protect the body from atherosclerotic cardiac disease. Fruits and vegetables are naturally also rich in cleansing fiber.

Nuts and seeds are rich in healthy (non-saturated) fats and more essential in vitamin E that protects against "bad" (saturated/trans fats. Nuts fill you and are a perfect choice for a balanced snack.

Foods To Avoid:

The fried foods are among the heart's worst foods. They are rich in cholesterol-related saturated fats. Most people were aware of the health dangers of fast food, but the food in the restaurant can be just as bad for you.

For a good cause, Red Meat has earned a poor reputation. The marbled cuts are worse and have a higher fat percentage. Try restricting your consumption to as much fat as you can once a week or less before cooking.

I assume most people are not shocked by the above guidance but have trouble applying these activities in their everyday lives. Here are some tips for a superfood that make it easy to eat healthily.

Purchase whole-grain cereals and bread.

Get to know safe recipes and try new stuff.

Replace butter or shortening with olive oil.

Leave on the counter new fruit.

Buy 1% milk or skim

The investigation is definitive. Hypertension and cholesterol have been correlated with our diet. Heart safe food is not rocket science, but some discipline is important. You can be shocked how easy it is to eat healthier, and thank you for your heart. Using the DASH diet to protect yourself against heart disease.

RECIPES

Berries Oatmeal with Honey
Ingredients:

- 1 Half mugs unsweetened plain almond milk
- One-Eighth tsp. vanilla extract
- 1 mug old-fashioned oats
- Third-Fourth mug combine of blueberries, blackberries, and coarsely Diced
- Strawberries
- 2 tbsps. Heat upped pecans
- Honey

Instructions:

- Heat up the almond milk and vanilla during a small dip saucepan on medium-sized Heat up. Once the mixture begins to simmer, add the oats and whisk for about four minutes, or until most of the liquid is absorbed.
- Whisk within the berries. Scoop the mixture into two dishes, and high with Heat upped pecans.

Banana and Apple Fritters
Ingredients:

- Half mug fat free milk
- 1 egg
- 1 tbsp. canola oil
- Half mug Diced banana
- Half mug Diced apple
- 1 mug whole warm up pastry flour
- 1 tbsp. (1 Half g) Lactose alternative,
- 1 tbsp. baking powder
- Half tsp. nutmegs

Instructions:

- Whisk along flour, Lactose various, and baking powder. Merge the milk, egg, and oil. Add banana, apple, and nutmeg. Whisk into dry ingredients, whisking until simply moistened.
- Drop by tubsful into warm oil. Fry for 2 to three minutes on a side till golden brown. Drain on paper towels before serving.

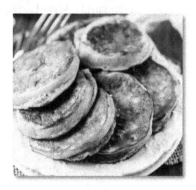

Orange Smoothie
Ingredients:

- 1 tsp. vanilla
- 2 ice cubes
- 1 Half mug (355 ml) buttermilk
- One-Third mug (83 g) orange juice concentrate
- 2 tbsps. brown Lactose

Instructions:

- In a blender canister, Merge buttermilk, orange juice concentrate, brown Lactose, and vanilla. Cover and blend until sleek. With blender running, add ice cubes piecemeal, through gap in lid. Blend till swish and frothy.

Banana and Blueberries Smoothie
Ingredients:

- 1 mug blueberries
- 2 mugs diced banana
- 2 mugs (460 g) low-fat peach curd

Instructions:

- Combine all ingredients in a blender. Add some water to make it thin. Serve immediately with honey.

Banana Curd Smoothie
Ingredients:

- 1 mug fat free milk
- 2 tbsps. curd (any flavor)
- 1 banana, broken in pieces
- 1 tsp. honey

Instructions:

- Put all ingredients in blender. Whip for 1 minute until smooth. Add ice cubes into blender to thicken, if you want. Serve immediately with honey.

Pineapple and Strawberry Smoothie
Ingredients:

- One-Fourth mug unsweetened pineapple juice
- Half mug frozen strawberries
- Half mug plain curd
- One-Fourth mug nonfat dry milk

Instructions:

- Blend all ingredients together in a blender. Transfer the mixture into cups. Serve immediately with honey.

Cinnamon Oat Baked Apple
Ingredients:

- 1 tbsp. pecans, coarsely Diced
- 1 tbsp. raisins
- One-Fourth tsp. cinnamon
- 4 apples, cored
- 4 ounces cheddar cheese
- 3 tbsps. quick Preparing oats
- 2 tbsps. brown Lactose
- 1 tbsp. oat bran
- Half mug cold mineral water

Instructions:

- Switch on oven to 375°F Cut half of cheese into small cubes; shred remainder. Combine cheese cubes, oats, brown Lactose, oat bran, pecans, raisins, and cinnamon till well blended. Put baking apples in square pan; fill with oat mixture. Spill mineral water in base of pan.
- Cover with foil; bake thirty minutes. Unwrap and continue baking 15 minutes or till ripe. Sprinkle with cut into tiny pieces cheese and continue baking till cheese is Defrosted.

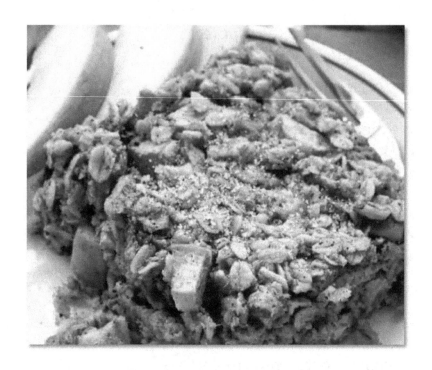

Pineapple Ham Boats
Ingredients:

- 2 tbsps. brown Lactose
- 1 tsp. poppy seeds
- Half-pound ham, thinly diced
- 2 pineapples
- 1 mug seedless green grapes
- 2 mugs bananas, diced
- One-Fourth pound Cheddar Cheese, chopped

Instructions:

- Slice pineapple longitudinally in half, crown to stem. Leave leafy crown on. Take away robust core. Loosen fruit by cutting to rind; cut in bite size pieces. Put in massive dish. Peel off bananas; slice. Cut grapes in half and boost pineapple.
- Roll with brown Lactose and poppy seeds. Line pineapple shells with ham. Serve fruit mixture on high. Prime with cheese.

Almond Butter and Banana
Ingredients:

- 1 small banana, diced
- One-Eighth tsp. ground cinnamon
- 2 slices 100% whole warm up bread
- 2 tbsps. almond butter

Instructions:

- Heat up the bread, and Expand each slice with almond butter. Sort the banana slices on Cover, and sprinkle with cinnamon. Serve immediately with honey.

Broccoli Garlic Omelet
Ingredients:

- 1 big clove garlic, minced
- One-Eighth tsp. chile pepper flakes
- One-Fourth mug low-fat feta cheese
- 2 egg whites
- 1 whole egg
- 2 tbsps. extra virgin olive oil
- Half mug Diced broccoli
- Cracked black pepper

Instructions:

- Whip the egg whites and egg in an exceedingly little dish. Warm up a tiny nonstick pan on medium-sized Warm up. Add 1 tbsp. of the oil to the new pan and when the oil is warm, add the broccoli. Prepare for 2 minutes before adding the garlic, chile pepper flakes, and black pepper to style. Prepare for two minutes more, then Take away the broccoli mixture from the pan, and Put in a very set apart dish.

- Flip the Warm up to low, add the left-over tbsp. of oil and when the oil is warm, add the Whipped eggs. Once they start to bubble and pull removed from the sides, regarding thirty seconds, flip the omelet over and instantly scoop the broccoli mixture and feta cheese on one half of the omelet.
- Fold the omelet over, flip off the Warm up, and cover the pan with a lid for 2 minutes. Serve instantly.

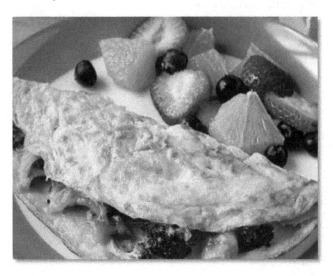

Strawberries Muffin with Berries
Ingredients:

- 4 strawberries, thinly diced
- Half mug blueberries, mashed
- 1 100% whole warm up English muffin, halved
- 1 tbsp. low-fat cream cheese

Instructions:

- Heat up the English muffin halves. Expand the cream cheese evenly on each Heat upped half, and Cover with the fruit.

Healthy Calories Free Muffin
Ingredients:

- 1 (4-ounce) can wild canned salmon in mineral water, no salt added, drained
- 6 thin slices unpeel offed cucumber
- 6 thin slices Roma tomato
- 1 100% whole warm up English muffin, halved
- One-Fourth tsp. finely Diced fresh dill
- Half tsp. fresh lemon juice
- 2 tbsps. low-fat cream cheese
- Cracked black pepper

Instructions:

- Heat up the English muffin halves. Meanwhile, during a tiny dish, combine the Diced dill and lemon juice evenly into the cream cheese. Expand the cream cheese mixture evenly onto every Heat upped muffin half.
- Soak the canned salmon below running mineral water to Take away the canned liquid, and then scoop the canned salmon evenly onto the English muffin halves. If the canned salmon is just too big, mash with fork initial. Cover with cucumber and tomato slices, and sprinkle with pepper to style.

Crustless Cheesy Quiche
Ingredients:

- 1 6 ounces cottage cheese
- 1 mug Cheddar Cheese cut into small pieces
- One-Third Mug Without salt butter
- Half mug ham, Diced
- 1 mug fat free milk
- 1 mug flour
- 6 eggs
- Half mug mushrooms, diced

Instructions:

- Switch on oven to 350°F. Combine all ingredients thoroughly except butter. Defrost butter and Spill half of it into a glass pan. Spill left-over butter into batter and Spill batter into pan. Bake for 50 minutes.

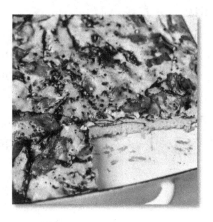

Energy Blueberries Oatmeal
Ingredients:

- 4 egg whites, Siren
- One-Eighth tsp. ground cinnamon
- One-Eighth tsp. ground ginger
- One-Fourth mug mineral water
- One-Fourth mug low-fat milk
- Half mug old-fashioned oats
- One-Fourth mug blueberries

Instructions:

- In a tiny pot, Warm up the mineral water and milk to a simmer on medium-sized Heat up. Add the oats, whisking constantly for concerning 4 minutes, or until most of the liquid is absorbed. Add the Siren egg whites slowly, whisking constantly.
- Prepare for an additional 5 minutes, or till the eggs are no longer runny. Whisk the cinnamon and ginger into the oatmeal mixture, and scoop the mixture into a dish. Cover with berries and serve instantly.

Coconut Barley with Berries
Ingredients:

- Half mug blackberries
- 2 tbsps. Heat upped Diced pecans
- 2 tsps. raw honey, optional
- 1 mug unprepared Barley
- 1 mug unsweetened coconut milk
- 1 mug mineral water

Instructions:

- Soak the Barley (if not presoaked). In a tiny Covered pot, bring the Barley, coconut milk and mineral water to a boil on high Warm up.
- Decrease the Warm up to low and simmer for 10 to fifteen minutes or until the liquid has been absorbed. ready Barley should be slightly al dente; it's ready when most of the grains have uncoiled and you can see the unwound germ. Let the Barley sit within the covered pot for regarding five minutes.
- Fluff gently with a fork and scoop into two dishes, and high with blackberries, pecans, and honey (if using).

Fruity Curd Parfait
Ingredients:

- One-Fourth mug chopped kiwifruit
- 1 tsp. ground flaxseeds or flaxseed meal
- Half mug low-calorie rolled oats, dry fruits, honey
- 1 mug low-fat plain Greek curd
- One-Fourth mug blueberries
- One-Fourth mug chopped strawberries

Instructions:

- Scoop half the curd into a small glass dish or parfait dish. Cover with a thin layer of blueberries, strawberries, kiwifruit, flaxseed meal, and rolled oats, dry fruits, honey.
- Layer the left-over curd and Cover with the left-over fruit, flaxseeds, and rolled oats, dry fruits, honey.

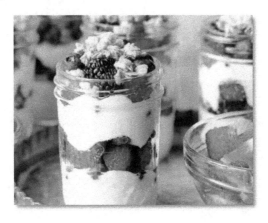

Banana Crunchy Almond Curd
Ingredients:

- One-Fourth mug unprepared old-fashioned oats
- Half big banana, diced
- 1 tbsp. raw, crunchy, Without salt almond butter
- Third-Fourth mug low-fat plain Greek curd
- One-Eighth tsp. ground cinnamon

Instructions:

- Soften the almond butter in the microwave for 15 seconds. Scoop the curd into a dish, and whisk in the almond butter, oats, and banana. Sprinkle cinnamon on Cover. Serve immediately.

Minced Veggie Frittata with Caramelized Onions
Ingredients:

- One-Fourth tsp. brown Lactose
- One-Eighth tsp. cracked black pepper
- 2–3 tbsps. extra virgin olive oil
- 1 Half mugs Diced cucumber
- 1 tbsp. extra-virgin olive oil
- 1 small white onion, thinly diced
- 1 clove garlic, minced
- 1 mug thinly diced cremini mushrooms
- 2–3 tbsps. finely Diced fresh basil
- Half mug cut into small pieces low-fat pepper jack cheese
- One-Eighth tsp. sea salt
- Cracked black pepper
- 1 tbsp. Diced fresh bay leaf or 1 tsp. parched bay leaf
- 2 mugs green lettuce
- 4 whole eggs
- 5 egg whites
- Half mug 1% milk

Instructions:

- Switch on the oven to 350°F. To caramelize the onions, Warm up a medium-sized dip saucepan over medium-sized Warm up. Add the oil and when the oil is warm, add the onion, Lactose, and pepper. Let the onion "sweat," moving it each couple of minutes to avoid burning, until light brown and softened, regarding ten minutes.
- Turn off the Warm up and cover the pan till ready to serve. Start the frittata by Warm upping a huge

pan over medium-sized Warm up and then adding the oil. Roll within the cucumber, and Prepare for concerning a minute. Add the garlic, and Prepare a pair of to three additional minutes before adding the mushrooms, basil, and bay leaf. Prepare veggies for another minute, sprinkle on salt and pepper (the mushrooms will unleash mineral water and cannot brown if you add the salt right away).

- Combine along, flip off the Warm up, and add the green lettuce. In a big dish, Whip together the eggs, egg whites, milk, cut into little items cheese, salt, and pepper. Sprinkle a nine-inch circular cake pan with olive oil Sprinkle. Spill in the Deep-fried ingredients and then the egg mixture. Put the pan on the middle rack of the oven, and Prepare for twenty to twenty-five minutes, or until a knife inserted in the middle comes out wipe.

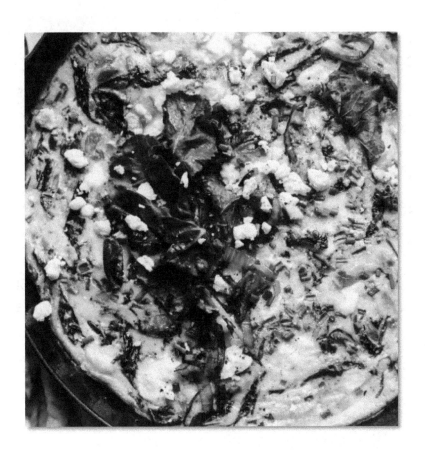

Egg Cheese Quiche
Ingredients:

- 8 ounces Cheddar Cheese, cut into small pieces
- One-Fourth mug parmesan cheese, grind
- 1 pie crust
- 1 mug cottage cheese
- 4 eggs, Siren

Instructions:

- Bake pie crust for 5 minutes at 425°F.
- Decrease temperature to 350°F (180°C). Combine ingredients and Spill into pie crust. Bake at 350°F for 45-50 minutes or until knife comes out wipe.

Garlic Veggie Scramble
Ingredients:

- 2 tbsps. extra virgin olive oil
- 2 tbsps. mineral water
- 1 big clove garlic, minced
- 3 whole eggs
- 1 mug combined greens (such as collard greens, mustard greens, and kale)
- One-Fourth mug Diced red onion
- One-Fourth mug Diced Poblano pepper
- Half mug Diced broccoli
- 3 egg whites
- One-Eighth tsp. sea salt
- Pinch of cracked black pepper

Instructions:

- Wash the greens and pat dry, bring to an end thick part of stems, and cut the leaves into items. Chop the onion, bell pepper, and broccoli into small pieces of concerning the same size. Warm up a huge nonstick frying pan over medium-sized to high Warm up and add the oil once the pan is warm. Add the greens once the oil is warm and Deep-fry for concerning 3 minutes or till the greens start to wilt.

- Spill the mineral water into the pan, cowl the pan with a lid, and Brew for 2 to 3 minutes. Take away the lid, add the broccoli, bell pepper, onion, and garlic. Meanwhile, in a very medium-sized dish, Whip along the eggs, egg whites, salt, and pepper. Once the onion is translucent, add the Whipped egg mixture. Whisk to evenly hack and distribute the eggs. Prepare till the eggs are not runny but still look a very little bit wet, turn off the Warm up, and serve instantly.

Cereal with Fruit
Ingredients:

- 1 orange, Peel offed and sectioned
- 3 One-Fourth mugs (765 ml) mineral water, Cut up
- Half mug Lactose alternative
- Half tsp. ground cinnamon
- 3 apples, Peel offed and thickly diced
- Half mug (88 g) prunes, pitted
- Third-Fourth mug raisins
- 2 tbsps. cornstarch
- 4 mugs rolled oats, dry fruits, honey

Instructions:

- In a dip saucepan, Merge apples, prunes, raisins, orange, and three mugs (70zero ml) mineral water. Bring to boil, decrease Heat up, and simmer 10 minutes. Whisk in Lactose different and cinnamon. Merge cornstarch and left-over mineral water.
- Whisk into dip saucepan. Prepare for 2 minutes. Serve over rolled oats, dry fruits, honey.

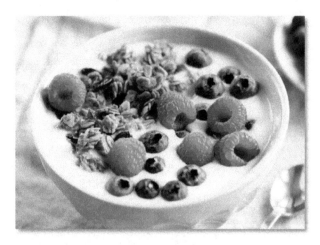

Mediterranean Scramble
Ingredients:

- One-Fourth mug diced Poblano pepper
- One-Fourth mug Soaked and drained, Diced canned artichoke hearts
- 2 egg whites
- 1 whole egg
- 2 tbsps. extra virgin olive oil
- One-Eighth mug Diced red onion
- 1 medium-sized clove garlic, minced
- One-Eighth tsp. parched oregano
- One-Eighth tsp. cracked black pepper
- One-Eighth mug low-fat feta cheese

Instructions:

- Warm up a small nonstick pan on medium-sized Warm up. Add oil to the warm pan and when the oil is warm, add the onion and garlic. Prepare for one minute before adding the bell pepper shreds and artichoke hearts.
- Deep-fry the veggies for one more 3 minute, or till the onion is translucent and therefore the bell pepper is softened. In a small dish, Whip the egg whites and egg, and season with oregano and black pepper. Spill the eggs in and mix them with a spatula. Prepare for 3 to four minutes, or until the eggs are now not runny. Take off from Warm up, high with feta, and cowl until the feta starts to Defrost. Serve instantly

Swiss Apple Panini
Ingredients:

- 8 slices whole-grain bread
- ¼ cup non-fat honey mustard
- 2 crisp apples, thinly sliced
- 6 oz. low-fat Swiss cheese, thinly sliced
- 1 cup arugula leaves
- Cooking spray

Instructions:

- Preheat your Panini press on a medium heat (Use a non-stick skillet if you do not own a Panini press)
- Spread a light coat of honey mustard over each slice of bread, evenly.
- Layer 4 slices of bread with the cheese, slices of apple and arugula leaves.
- Top each of these slices of bread with the remaining slices of bread.
- Coat your Panini press lightly with cooking spray.
- Grill sandwiches till the cheese melts and the bread has toasted. (Approx. 3 to 5 minutes)
- Remove the sandwiches from the press/ non-stick skillet.
- Allow sandwiches to cool slightly before serving them.

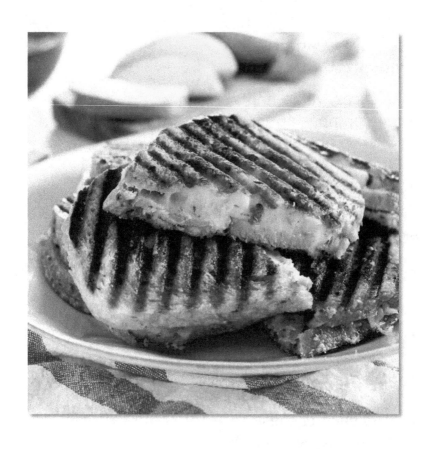

Vegetarian Pasta Soup
Ingredients:

- 2 tsps. olive oil
- 6 cloves garlic, minced
- 1 1/2 cups coarsely shredded carrot 1 cup chopped onion
- 1 cup thinly sliced celery
- 1 32-oz. box reduced-sodium chicken broth
- 4 cups water
- 1 1/2 cups dried ditalini pasta 1/4 cup shaved Parmesan cheese
- 2 Tbsps. snipped fresh parsley.

Instructions:

- Heat the olive oil in a 5-to 6-quart Dutch oven, over a medium heat.
- Add garlic to the pan and cook for 15 seconds.
- Add the shredded carrot, chopped onion and sliced celery to the pan and cook for a few minutes, stirring occasionally, until tender. (Approx. 5 to 7 minutes)
- Add the water and chicken broth to the pan and bring it to a boil.
- Add the uncooked pasta and cook until pasta is tender. (Approx. 7 to 8 minutes)
- Top each individual serving with Parmesan cheese and parsley when serving.

Grilled Veggie Toast Californian-Style
Ingredients:

- 3 Tbsps. light mayonnaise
- 3 cloves garlic, minced
- 1 Tbsp. lemon juice
- 1/8 cup olive oil
- 1 cup red bell peppers, sliced
- 1 small zucchini, sliced
- 1 red onion, sliced
- 1 small yellow squash, sliced
- 2 slices whole wheat focaccia bread
- ½ cup crumbled reduced-fat feta cheese

Instructions:

- Mix the lemon juice, mayonnaise and minced garlic in a bowl; refrigerate.
- Preheat grill on a high heat.
- Brush each side of vegetables with olive oil.
- Brush the grate of the grill with oil and place the zucchini and bell peppers in the middle of the grill, and set the sliced squash and onions around them.
- Grill for 3 minutes, turn, and grill for another 3 minutes. (Peppers might take longer to cook)
- Remove from heat and set aside.
- Spread the mayonnaise mix on the 2 slices of bread and sprinkle with feta cheese.
- Place the slices of bread on the grill, cheese side up, and cover for a few minutes. (Approx. 3 minutes)

- Check often to make sure the bottom does not burn.
- Remove the slices of bread from the grill and layer with vegetables.

Tuna Salad Tuscan-Style
Ingredients:

- 2 6-oz. cans chunk light tuna, drained 1 15-oz. can small white beans, such as cannellini or great northern 10 cherry tomatoes, quartered 4 scallions, trimmed and sliced
- 2 Tbsps. extra-virgin olive oil 2 Tbsps. lemon juice 1/4 tsp. salt
- Freshly ground pepper, to taste

Instructions:

- Add the tuna, scallions, beans, tomatoes, lemon juice, oil, salt and pepper to a medium bowl and stir gently.
- Refrigerate until you are ready to serve.

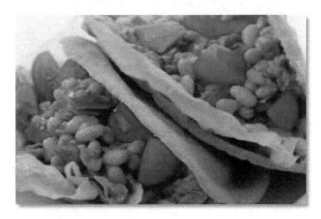

Tuna Melt English Muffins
Ingredients:

- 6 oz. white tuna
- packed in water, drained
- 1/3 cup chopped celery
- 1/4 cup chopped onion
- 1/4 cup low fat Russian or Thousand Island salad dressing
- 2 whole-wheat English muffins, split
- 3 oz. reduced-fat Cheddar cheese, grated
- Salt and black pepper to taste

INSTRUCTIONS:

- Preheat broiler
- Mix the tuna, celery, onion and salad dressing in a bowl and season it with salt and pepper.
- Toast the split English muffins and place them on a baking sheet, split-side-up.
- Top each muffin half with ¼ of the tuna mix.
- Broil the muffins until heated through. (Approx. 2 to 3 minutes)
- Top the muffins with cheese and return to broiler.
- Broil until cheese is melted. (Approx. 1 minute)

Delightful Tortellini Salad
Ingredients:

- 1 9-oz. package refrigerated light cheese tortellini or ravioli
- 3 cups broccoli florets
- 1 cup crinkle-cut or sliced carrots (2 medium) 1/4 cup sliced green onions (2)
- 1/2 cup bottled reduced-fat ranch salad dressing 1 large tomato, chopped
- 1 cup fresh pea pods, halved
- Milk (optional)

Instructions:

- Cook pasta in a large saucepan according to the Instructions on the package.
- Add the sliced carrots and broccoli during the last 3 minutes of boiling.
- Drain, rinse the cooked pasta and vegetables with cold water, and drain again.
- Combine the cooked pasta mix and green onions in a large bowl, drizzle with dressing, and gently toss to coat.
- Cover and chill for at least 2 hours.
- Gently stir in the tomato and pea pods into the pasta mix before serving.
- Stir in a little milk to moisten if necessary.

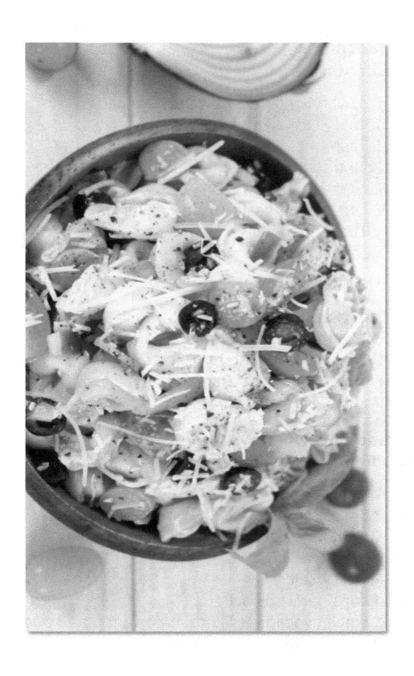

Healthy Tuna Salad
Ingredients:

- 5 oz can light tuna in water, drained
- 1 Tbsp. extra-virgin olive oil
- 1 Tbsp. red wine vinegar
- ¼ cup chopped green onion tops
- 2 cups arugula
- 1 cup cooked pasta (from 2 oz dry)
- 1 Tbsp. fresh shaved parmesan cheese
- black pepper

Instructions:

- Add the tuna, oil, vinegar, arugula, onion and cooked pasta in a large bowl and toss.
- Divide the mix onto two plates.
- Garnish with parmesan and pepper, and serve immediately.

Avocado, Strawberry & Melon Salad
Ingredients:

- 1/4 cup honey
- 2 Tbsps. sherry vinegar, or red-wine vinegar 2 Tbsps. finely chopped fresh mint
- 1/4 tsp. freshly ground pepper
- Pinch of salt
- 4 cups baby spinach
- 1 small avocado, (4-5 oz.), peeled, pitted and cut into 16 slices 16 thin slices
- cantaloupe, (about 1/2 small cantaloupe), rind removed 1 1/2 cups hulled
- strawberries, sliced

- 2 tsps. sesame seeds, toasted

Instructions:

- Add honey, vinegar, fresh mint, pepper and salt to a small bowl and whisk.
- Divide the baby spinach equally onto 4 plates.
- Arrange the slices of avocado and cantaloupe in a fan on top of the spinach, alternatively.
- Top each salad with strawberries and drizzle it with the honey dressing.
- Sprinkle sesame seeds on top and serve.

Cheesy Pear & Turkey Sandwich
Ingredients:

- 2 slices whole wheat bread
- 2 tsp Dijon-style mustard
- 2 slices (1 oz. each) reduced-sodium cooked or smoked turkey
- 1 USA pear, cored and thinly sliced
- 1/4 cup shredded low fat mozzarella cheese
- Coarsely ground pepper

Instructions:

- Spread a tsp. of mustard on both slices of bread.
- Place a slice of turkey on each slice of bread and arrange the slices of pair on top.
- Sprinkle both slices of bread with 2 Tbsps. of cheese and pepper.
- Broil it 4 to 6 inches from heat until turkey and pears are warm and cheese has melted. (Approx. 2 to 3 minutes) Cut sandwiches in half.
- Serve open face.

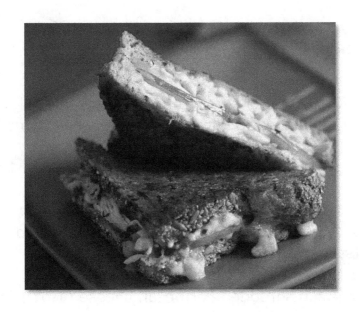

Chunky Tomato Spaghetti Squash
Ingredients:

- 1 lb. lean ground beef
- 1/2 cup chopped onion (1 medium)
- 1/2 cup chopped green sweet pepper (1 small) 2 cloves garlic, minced
- 1 14 1/2-oz. can dice tomatoes, undrained 1 8-oz. can tomato sauce
- 2 Tbsps. tomato paste
- 1-1/2 tsps. dried Italian seasoning, crushed 1/8 tsp. black pepper
- 1 recipe Cooked Spaghetti Squash
- 1/4 cup shredded Parmesan cheese (1 oz.) Small fresh basil leaves (optional)

Instructions:

- Cook the ground beef, sweet pepper, onion and garlic in a large saucepan until the meat turns brown; drain.
- Add the undrained diced tomato, tomato paste, tomato sauce, Italian seasoning and black pepper and bring the sauce to a boil.
- Reduce heat and simmer, uncovered for 14 to 16 minutes; stir occasionally.
- In the meantime, prepare the Cooked Spaghetti Squash.
- Serve the sauce over the Squash and sprinkle parmesan cheese on top.
- Garnish with basil leaves if desired.
- Use a sharp knife to prick the Squash in a few places.

- Place the Squash in a microwave-safe baking dish and microwave uncovered on high power (100%) until tender. (Approx. 10 to 15 minutes) • Let stand for 4 to 6 minutes.
- Cut the squash into 2 halves, lengthwise and remove seeds.
- Shred and separate the squash pulp into strands using 2 forks.

Pita-Pizza
Ingredients:

- 2 pieces whole wheat pita bread
- ½ cup grated reduced sodium mozzarella cheese
- ¼ cup pizza or tomato sauce
- Veggies of choice: mushrooms, bell pepper, onion, olives, artichoke hearts, etc.

Instructions:

- Preheat toaster or oven to 350 degrees.
- Split the 2 pieces of pita bread halfway around the edge, and spoon in the cheese, tomato sauce and any topping of your choice.
- Wrap the pita bread in aluminum foil.
- Bake for a few minutes until cheese has melted. (Approx. 7 to 10 minutes)

Mushroom, Tofu & Spinach Soba Noodles Mix
Ingredients:

- 2 Tbsp. (30 mL) canola oil
- 1 shallot, minced
- 1 carrot, finely diced
- 2 cloves garlic, minced
- 1-1/2 Tbsp. (20 mL) minced fresh ginger
- 8 oz. (250 g) white or brown mushrooms, sliced 1 cup (250 mL) frozen,
- thawed edamame
- 1-1/2 cups (375 mL) low-sodium chicken broth or vegetable broth 2 Tbsp.
- (30 mL) reduced-sodium soy sauce
- 1 tsp. (5 mL) grated lemon zest
- 4 oz. (125 g) spinach leaves, chopped
- 4 oz. (125 g) firm tofu, cut into 1/2-inch dice 1/4 tsp. (1 mL) freshly ground
- pepper
- 6 oz. (170 g) soba noodles

Instructions:

- Boil a 5 to 6-quart pot of water.
- Warm the canola oil in a 10-inch sauté pan over a medium-high heat.
- Add the diced carrots, ginger and garlic, and sauté for about a minute.
- Stir in the mushrooms and reduce heat to low.
- Cover the pan and sweat mushrooms until they are tender. (Approx. 4 minutes)
- Uncover the pan and increase heat back to a medium-high setting.

- Stir in the edamame and sauté until it is heated through. (Approx. 2 minutes)
- Stir the broth, lemon zest and soy sauce together.
- Pour it into the pan and bring it to a boil.
- Stir in the spinach, only a handful at a time, stirring after each addition until the leaves wilt.
- Add the tofu, stir it in, and turn off the heat.
- Season with pepper.
- Drop the soba noodles into the boiling pot of water and cook. (Approx. 5 minutes)
- Drain the pasta in a colander and rinse using cold water to remove excess starch.
- Add the soba noodles to the sauté pan and return to a medium-high heat.
- Toss noodles with a pair of tongs and mix with the vegetables until heated through.
- Divide and serve among pasta bowls.

Salmon Salad in a Pita
Ingredients:

- ¾ cup canned Alaskan
- salmon
- 3 Tbsps. plain fat-free yogurt
- 1 Tbsp. lemon juice
- 2 Tbsps. red bell pepper, minced
- 1 Tbsp. red onion, minced
- 1 tsp. capers, rinsed and chopped
- Pinch of dill, fresh or dried
- Black pepper to taste
- 3 lettuce leaves
- 3 pieces small whole wheat pita bread

Instructions:

- Mix the salmon, fat-free yogurt, lemon juice, red bell pepper, red onion, capers, dill and black pepper in a bowl to make the salmon salad.
- Place a lettuce leaf and 1/3 cup of the salmon salad inside each pita.

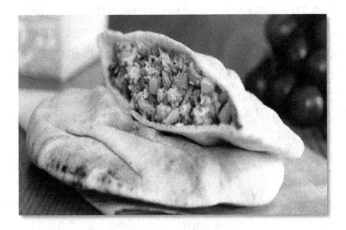

Skillet Potatoes and Sausage
Ingredients:

- 1/2 lb. cooked smoked low sodium turkey sausage 3 to 4 Tbsps. olive oil or
- cooking oil 1-3/4 lbs. unpeeled red-skinned potatoes
- 2 medium onions
- 1 tsp. dried thyme, crushed
- 1-1/2 to 2 tsps. cumin seed, slightly crushed 1/4 tsp. salt
- 1/4 tsp. pepper

Instructions:

- Pack ingredients to transport; pack sausages in an insulated cooler with ice picks to transport.
- Pour 3 Tbsps. of olive oil (or cooking oil) into a 10-inch, heavy, ovenproof skillet.
- Tilt skillet to coat the bottom of the skillet with oil.
- Place directly over campfire.
- Cut the potatoes into ½ inch cubes.
- Chop the onions or slice into thin wedges.
- Add the potatoes and onions to the hot oil and cook uncovered on a medium high heat, stirring occasionally until potatoes are near tender. (Approx. 12 to 13 minutes)
- Slice the sausages diagonally and add to the potato mix.
- If necessary, add a Tbsp. of oil to prevent sticking.
- Cook uncovered until potatoes and onions are fully tender and slightly golden; stir often.

- Stir in the cumin seed, thyme, salt and pepper.
- Cook for about a minute more.

Rice Bowl, Southwest-Style
Ingredients:

- 1 tsp. vegetable oil
- 1 cup chopped vegetables (try a mixture - bell peppers, onion, corn, tomato,
- zucchini)
- 1 cup cooked meat (chopped or shredded)
- 1 cup cooked brown rice
- 4 Tbsps. salsa
- 2 Tbsps. shredded cheese
- 2 Tbsps. Low Fat Sour Cream

Instructions:

- Heat oil over medium high heat in a medium skillet. (350 degrees if an electric skillet) • Add the vegetables and cook until vegetables are tender-crisp. (Approx. 3 to 5 minutes) • Add the cooked meat, beans or tofu and cooked rice to the skillet and heat it through.
- Divide the rice mix between 2 bowls.
- Top each serving with salsa, cheese and sour cream.
- Serve warm.
- Refrigerate leftovers within 2 hours.

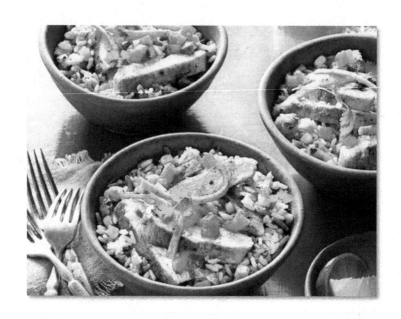

Sirloin Potage
Ingredients:

- 1 Tbsp. oil
- 1 small onion, diced
- 1 lb. lean ground sirloin
- 1/3 cup all-purpose flour
- 1 package (32 oz.) beef broth
- 1 bag (1 lb.) frozen soup vegetables 2 Tbsps. Worcestershire sauce

Instructions:

- Heat the oil in a large saucepan over medium heat.
- Add the diced onion and cook for a few minutes until onions are soft.
- Add the ground beef and cook while breaking up chunks with a spoon, till it is cooked through. (Approx. 5 minutes)
- In a jar with a tight-fitting lid, place the flour and 2/3 cup of water and shake to blend well.
- Pour the mix into the saucepan with beef and add the beef broth.
- Bring it to a boil while stirring constantly.
- Add the vegetables and simmer until cooked. (Approx. 10 minutes)
- Add the Worcestershire sauce to the saucepan and stir it in.
- Serve while hot.

Shrimp, Corn & Raspberry Salad
Ingredients:

- 12 oz. fresh asparagus spears
- 1 8-oz. package frozen baby corn or 8-3/4-oz. can baby corn, drained 12
- Belgian endive leaves or curly endive leaves 12 Boston or Bibb lettuce leaves
- 12 sorrel or spinach leaves
- 12 oz. fresh or frozen peeled and deveined shrimp, cooked and chilled 2-1/2
- cups fresh or frozen red raspberries and/or sliced strawberries, thawed 1/4
- cup walnut oil or salad oil
- 1/4 cup raspberry or wine vinegar
- 1 Tbsp. snipped fresh cilantro or parsley 2 tsps. honey

Instructions:

- Discard the woody bases of the asparagus by snapping it off.
- Cover the asparagus in a small amount of boiling water and cook until it is crisp-tender. (Approx. 4 to 8 minutes)
- Drain and leave to cool.
- If you are using frozen baby corn, cook according to the Instructions on the package.
- Drain and leave to cool.
- Arrange the asparagus and greens on 4 dinner plates, and top each with shrimp, corn and berries.
- For salad dressing; combine walnut oil or salad oil, wine or raspberry vinegar, parsley or fresh

cilantro and honey in a screw-top jar, cover, and shake well.
- Serve the dressing with the salad.

Black Bean and Guacamole Cake, Southwestern-Style

Ingredients:

- 2 slices whole wheat bread, torn
- 3 Tbsps. fresh cilantro
- 2 cloves garlic
- 1 (15-oz.) can low sodium black beans, rinsed and drained
- 1 (7-oz.) can chipotle peppers in adobo sauce
- 1 tsp. ground cumin
- 1 large egg
- ½ medium avocado, seeded and peeled
- 1 Tbsp. lime juice
- 1 small plum tomato

Instructions:

- Add the corn bread into a food processor, cover and blend until the bread resembles grainy crumbs.
- Transfer the crumbs to a large bowl and set it aside.
- Blend the cilantro and garlic until they are finely chopped.
- Add 1 chipotle pepper, beans, 1 ½ tsps. of adobo sauce and cumin to blender and blend using the on/ off pulse until beans are chopped and the mix starts to pull away from the sides.
- Add the mix to the bowl of bread crumbs.
- Add an egg and mix.
- Shape the mixture into four patties of ½ inch thickness.

- Grill the patties on a lightly greased grill rack, over a medium heat until both sides of the patties are heated through. (Approx. 8 minutes)
- In the meantime, for the guacamole, mash avocado in a small bowl and stir in the lime juice.
- Season it with salt and pepper.
- Serve the patties with tomato and guacamole.

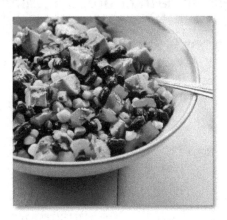

Cheesy Mushroom & Spinach Wraps
Ingredients:

- 1 Tbsp. olive oil
- 8 oz. fresh mushrooms, sliced (about 2 ½ cups)
- 1 tsp. minced garlic
- 2 whole wheat 8" tortillas
- ½ lb. fresh spinach or arugula, trimmed and steamed
- 1 plum tomato, diced
- ¼ Cup (1 Oz.) Shredded Part-Skim Mozzarella Cheese

Instructions:

- Preheat oven to 350ºF.
- In a sauté pan, heat a Tbsp. of olive oil over a high heat.
- Add a layer of garlic and mushroom and let sauté; be patient till the mushrooms turn a red-brown color, then turn over and sauté until it turns a similar color.
- Arrange the spinach in layers over each tortilla, and add the cooked mushrooms, tomato and mozzarella on top.
- Roll up the tortillas.
- Slightly oil a baking dish and place the tortillas seam-side down.
- Bake until the cheese melts. (Approx. 10 minutes)
  • Cut the tortillas into quarters, crosswise.
- Serve while warm.

Taco Chicken Salad
Ingredients:

- 1/3 cup chopped or shredded cooked chicken or low sodium turkey 2 Tbsps.
- chopped celery
- 1 Tbsp. light mayonnaise dressing or salad dressing 1 Tbsp. salsa
- 1 Tbsp. shredded cheddar cheese
- 4 Mini taco shells or scoop-shaped tortilla chips

Instructions:

- For chicken salad; combine chicken, celery, mayonnaise dressing, salsa and cheese in a small bowl and toss to mix.
- Spoon the salad into a container and cover tightly.
- Wrap taco shells in a plastic wrap and pack both chicken salad and taco shells into an insulated bag with an ice pack.
- When serving, use the taco shells to scoop up the salad.

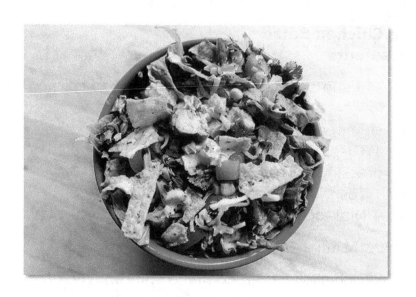

Sunshine in A Wrap
Ingredients:

- 8 oz chicken breast (one large breast)
- ½ cup celery, diced
- 2/3 cup canned mandarin oranges, drained
- ¼ cup onion, minced
- 2 Tbsps. mayonnaise
- 1 tsp. soy sauce
- ¼ tsp. garlic powder
- ¼ tsp. black pepper
- 1 large whole wheat tortilla
- 4 Large Lettuce Leaves, Washed and Patted Dry

Instructions:

- Cook the chicken breast in a non-stick pan over a medium-high heat; cook until heated through.
- Remove from heat and once chicken has cooled, cut into small cubes.
- Mix the chicken, oranges, celery and onions in a medium bowl.
- Add soy sauce, garlic, mayonnaise and pepper, and mix well until the chicken is evenly coated.
- Lay a tortilla on a cutting board and cut into 4 quarters.
- Place a lettuce leaf on each quarter and trim the parts of the lettuce leaf that hang over the tortilla.
- Divide the chicken mix evenly between the tortilla quarters and place in the middle of each lettuce leaf.

- Roll the quarters into a cone; the 2 straight edges coming together while the curved edge creates the opening of the cone.
- Serve as a sandwich wrap.
- Refrigerate the leftovers within 2 hours of preparing.

Quesadillas & Cilantro-Yogurt Dip
Ingredients:

- 1 cup beans, black or pinto
- 2 Tbsps. cilantro, chopped
- ½ bell pepper, finely chopped
- ½ cup corn kernels
- 1 cup low-fat shredded cheese
- 6 soft corn tortillas
- 1 medium carrot, shredded
- ½ jalapeno pepper, finely minced (optional)
  CILANTRO YOGURT DIP:
- 1 cup plain non-fat yogurt
- 2 Tbsps. cilantro, finely chopped
- Juice from ½ of a lime

Instructions:

- Preheat a large skillet over a low heat.
- Line up 3 tortillas and divide the cheese, beans, corn, shredded carrots, cilantro and peppers between them.
- Cover each tortilla with a second tortilla and place each tortilla on a dry skillet and warm until cheese has melted and tortilla is slightly golden. (Approx. 3 minutes)
- Flip the tortillas and cook the other side until slightly golden. (Approx. 1 minute) • Mix the nonfat yogurt, cilantro and lime juice in a small bowl.
- Cut each of the quesadillas into 4 wedges (for a total of 12 wedges.) • Serve 3 wedges per person with 1/4 cup of the dip.
- Refrigerate the leftovers within 2 hours.

Roast Chicken Dahl Curry
Ingredients:

- 1 1/2 tsps. canola oil
- 1 small onion, minced
- 2 tsps. curry powder
- 1 15-oz. can lentils, rinsed, or 2 cups cooked lentils 1 14-oz. can diced
- tomatoes, preferably fire-roasted 1 2-lb. roasted chicken, skin discarded, meat
- removed from bones and diced (4 cups) 1/4 tsp. salt, or to taste
- 1/4 cup low-fat plain yogurt

Instructions:

- In a heavy, large saucepan, heat the oil over a medium-high heat.
- Add the onion to the saucepan and stir until soft, but not browned. (Approx. 3 to 4 minutes) • Stir in the curry powder and cook until it is combined with the onion and is intensely aromatic. (Approx. 20 to 30 seconds)
- Add the chicken, tomatoes, lentils and salt.
- Cook while stirring often until it is heated through.
- Remove saucepan from the heat and stir in the yogurt.
- Serve while hot.

Apple Turkey Wrap
Ingredients:

- 1 Tbsp. vegetable oil
- 1 cup onion, sliced
- 1 cup sweet red pepper, thinly sliced
- 1 cup sweet green pepper, thinly sliced
- 2 Tbsps. lemon juice
- ½ lb. cooked low sodium turkey or chicken breast, cut into thin strips
- 1 Golden Delicious apple, cored and finely chopped
- 6 whole wheat pocket pita bread, warmed
- ½ cup low fat or fat free plain yogurt

Instructions:

- Heat the vegetable oil over medium heat in a large skillet.

- Once oil is heated, add the sliced onion, pepper and lemon juice; cook until it is tender.
- Add the turkey and apple to the skillet and cook until the turkey is heated through.
- Remove from heat and fill each pita with some of this mix.
- Drizzle each pita with yogurt.
- Serve warm.

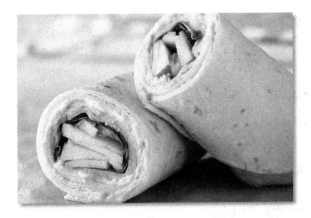

Ketchup & Mustard Glazed Pork Ribs
Ingredients:

- 1 rack pork ribs, cut into individual ribs, about 3 lbs.
- 1-1/4 cups ketchup
- 1/3 cup cider vinegar
- 3 Tbsps. spicy brown mustard 2 Tbsps. brown sugar
- 3 Tbsps. water
- 1 tsp. onion powder
- 1/4 Tsp. Hot Sauce

Instructions:

- Heat oven to 400°F.
- Place the pork ribs in a 13 x 9 x 2-dimension baking dish and cover with foil.
- Bake for an hour at 400°F.
- Drain the liquid.
- In the meantime, stir the mustard, ketchup, brown sugar, vinegar, onion powder, hot sauce and water together in a medium-size saucepan.
- Cook, while stirring over a medium-low heat.
- Place half of the sauce in a bowl and set aside.
- Heat your grill to a medium high heat and lightly coat grill rack with oil.
- Baste the pork ribs with the remaining sauce generously and grill for 4 minutes per side until the meat has browned well.
- Serve the pork ribs with the balance sauce on the side.

Amazing Cucumber Salad
Ingredients:

- 24 cherry tomatoes
- 1 Half mugs cucumber, diced
- Half mug white lemon juice
- 9 mugs romaine green lettuce leaf, torn into bite-sized pieces
- 4 ounces salami
- 1 mug carrot, diced
- One-Fourth mug green olives, diced
- 8 ounces mushrooms, diced
- 1 mug red onion, diced
- 12 ounces tuna, mineral water packed
- 6 tbsps. Parmesan cheese, grind
- 10 ounces frozen green beans, prepared and cooled
- 2 mugs garbanzo beans
- 8 ounces roasted red pepper
- 2 tbsps. olive oil
- 3 ounces (85 g) no-salt-added tomato paste
- 4 ounces pimento

Instructions:

- Merge lemon juice, olive oil, and tomato paste in a dip saucepan and Warm up over medium-sized Warm up until warm and well Merged. Take away and let cool. Cut veggies into bite-sized pieces and augment the cooled mixture.
- Add garbanzo beans and whisk to Merge. Cut up inexperienced lettuce leaf among serving plates

and Cover with vegetable mixture, meat, and fish. Sprinkle with the Parmesan cheese.

Beef and Barley Salad
Ingredients:

- 1 clove garlic, minced
- 1-ounce sesame seeds
- 8 ounces leftover roast beef
- Half-pound green lettuce leaf, cut into small pieces
- Half tsp. ground ginger
- 1 tbsp. Lactose
- 1 mug carrot, diced
- 2 mugs (314 g) prepared barley
- 8 ounces snow peas
- 8 ounces mushrooms, diced
- 1 mug Poblano pepper, diced
- 4 ounces mung bean sprouts
- One-Fourth mug balsamic lemon juice
- 2 tbsps. sesame oil
- 1 mug cabbage, cut into small pieces

Instructions:

- Merge marinade ingredients. Slice beef and Put in a plastic baggie with marinade for 1 to 2 hours. Drain, reserving liquid. Roll salad ingredients and Cover with beef slices.
- Serve left-over dressing over Cover.

Dinner Poblano pepper Salad
Ingredients:

- 2 tbsps. red wine lemon juice
- 4 mugs (188 g) romaine green lettuce leaf, finely Diced
- 2 mugs cabbage, finely Diced

- 1 mug Poblano pepper, Diced
- 1 mug Poblano pepper, Diced
- 4 ounces black olives
- Half mug celery, thinly diced
- 2 mugs garbanzo beans, drained
- One-Fourth mug olive oil
- 1 tsp. balsamic lemon juice
- Half tsp. garlic, minced
- 1 tsp. lemon juice
- 1 tbsp. Spicy Brown Mustard
- 1 tsp. Lactose
- 4 ounces dry salami, cut up
- 4 ounces Cheddar Cheese, cut up
- 6 ounces boneless chicken breast, prepared and Diced
- One-Eighth tsp. black pepper, fresh ground

Instructions:

- Cut up green lettuce leaf between 6 plates. Sort other veggies, meats, and cheese over green lettuce leaf. Shake dressing ingredients together and Sprinkle over salads. Serve immediately.

CPSIA information can be obtained
at www.ICGtesting.com
Printed in the USA
BVHW092201220421
605633BV00004B/615